Essential Oil Recipes

For Weight Loss

Relaxing Your Way to Fitness

Disclaimer

Summary

Did you believe essential oils are just pleasantly scented compounds that can be used as perfumes? Well, your perception about essential oils is about to be destroyed!

You will find a whole new perspective to the uses of essential oils – as scented extracts, edibles and topical applications as well. Essential oils can be rightly used to promote weight loss and achieve a fit physique. In this book you will find:

1. The basic definition of essential oils
2. The list of benefits attached with their usage
3. A detailed analysis of whether essential oils can promote weight loss or not
4. The role of essential oils in weight loss
5. The different ways in which essential oils can be used for weight loss
6. 50 distinct recipes using essential oils to help in weight loss
7. And lots more!

Explore this world of massive potential and turn the tables in your favor. Your dream physique need not remain a dream. Everything you need to know about the use of essential oils for weight loss is contained in here!

So what are you waiting for? Grab a copy today and approach your fitness goals in a way that yields guaranteed results!

Contents

Introduction

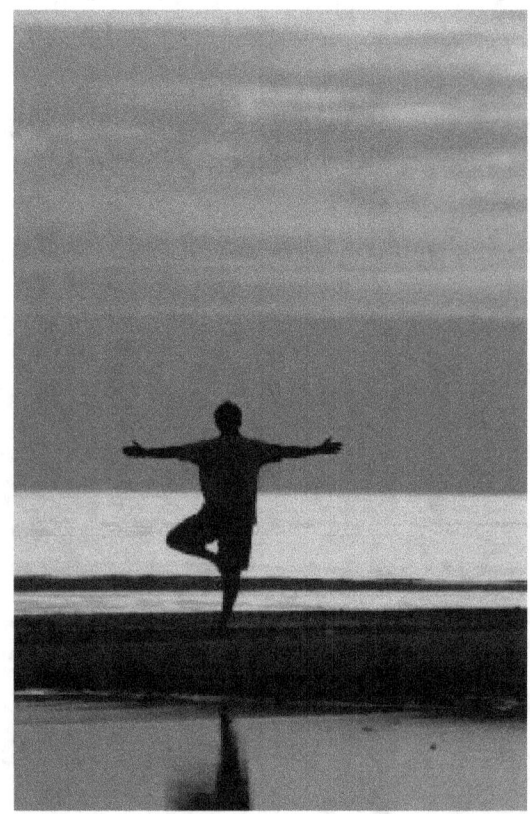

Everyone likes being praised for picture perfect physiques. It is one thing that is within your sphere of control yet tends to be taken as a major challenge. Your cravings to try out different cuisines are likely to be the culprit behind your sense of hopelessness. After all, when there are so many delicacies to try out, who would be bothered about health and fitness?

This results in gradual aggravation which ultimately raises alarms at some point in time. At this stage, quite a few otherwise effective recipes become useless because there is simply too much fat to cut down. You try out one weight loss regime after another only to find there is no viable solution to your cravings. But that was before you came across this recipe book!

Essential oils can help you lose weight. There are a number of ways you can bring them into use. But first things first; what are essential oils?

What are Essential Oils?

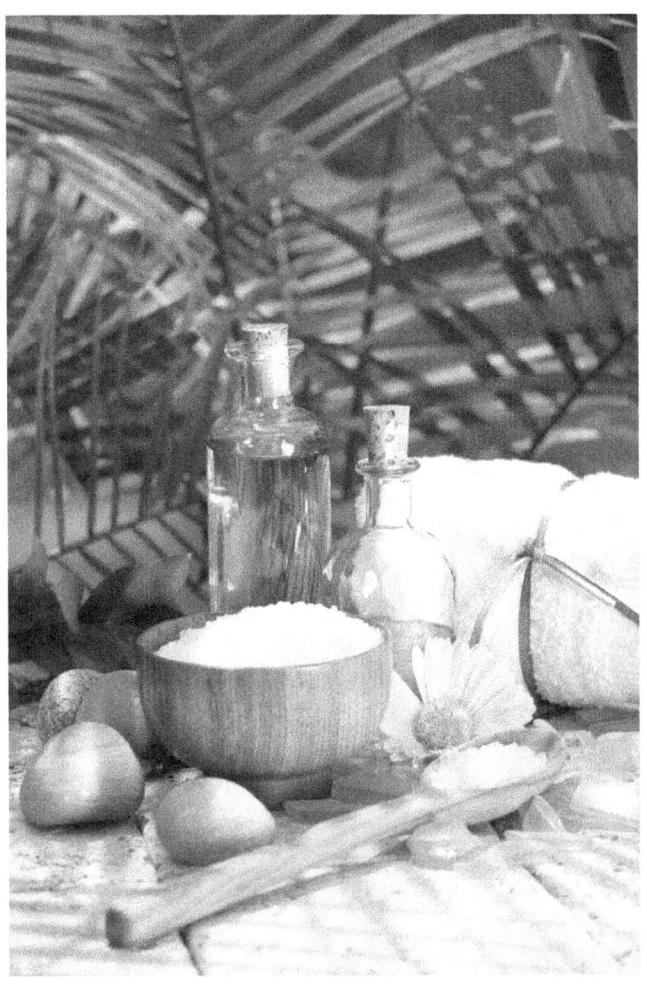

Simply put, essential oils are extracts. They can be retrieved from flowers, leaves, wood, bark, roots, seeds or peals. It involves a complex distillation process in which the "essence" of the plant is preserved in the form of a pure liquid.

The essential oils are known to have a distinctive smell typical for the plant they have been extracted from. They are usually volatile and will evaporate readily – and hence allowing the scent to reach you. This is why essential oils have been popularly used as perfumes for centuries.

Essential oils, until the past century, were simply scented liquid. They were to be mixed in specific proportions to create unique and even more exotic smells. It is typical for women to use these elements of nature; however, it is not uncommon for men to use these secret concoctions either nowadays.

Essential oils can be used for a number of reasons. The first and foremost, as obvious from its very nature, is its use as a perfume. Furthermore, certain essential oils are known to have medicinal properties as well. Hence their usage in medicines and pharmacological products is also quite common. Moreover, they can be used for personal grooming as an unparalleled skincare product.

They are not essential for health but are known to have a positive impact thereof. The clear liquid of essential oils is nothing short of a miracle – which you will well administer once you have read through this eBook. Keep reading to find out everything about this miracle of nature!

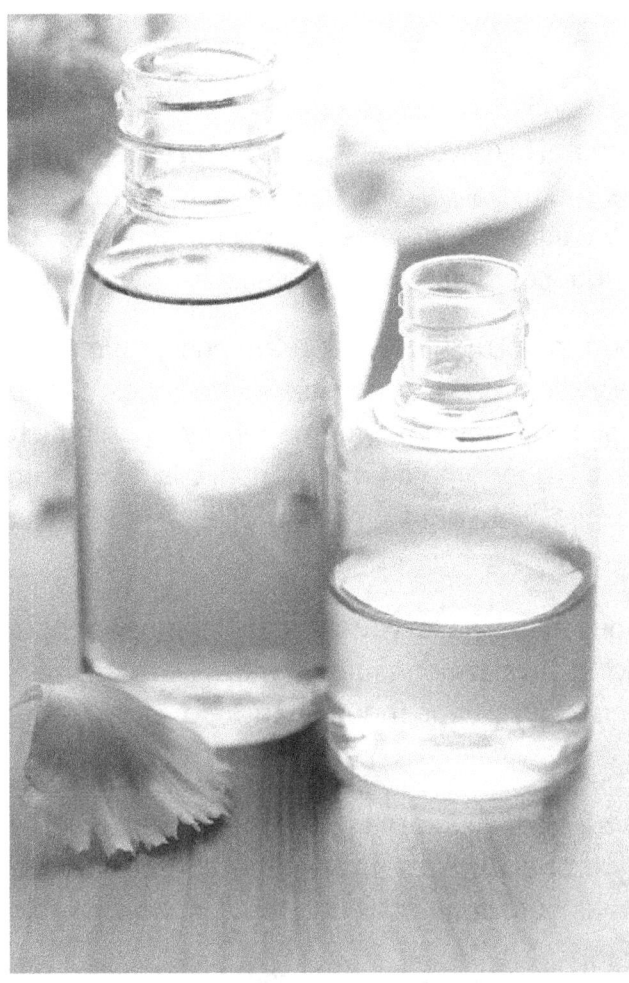

It is actually the crux of the story – do essential oils really help in losing weight? It has been a well debated topic for quite a few years now. There is no doubt about the medicinal and health benefits of using essential oils but when you are focused around a specific purpose, the scenario is a little different.

Essential oils do help in weight loss but they work differently. Here is a little insight to the topic to help you understand the procedure in a better way.

Essential oils are used in a number of ways for weight loss. For instance, it can be applied externally on your body, can be ingested, inhaled or used for soaking and bathing. The way each mode of use affects your body is different. However, the right use of essential oils can help you achieve your fitness motives.

When you feel excessive cravings for foods, inhaling certain essential oils is known to help alleviate these hunger pangs. The scent influences your brain to perceive satisfaction even without consuming anything. This helps you in keeping excess calories at bay by remaining faithful with your diet plan. The best part about this is that the influence is natural and not chemical – so there are no side effects known to affect your health.

Moreover, when the essential oil is consumed orally, the effect is seen in the form of higher metabolism rates. This eventually burns more calories so you can get rid of excess body fat. Once the readily available energy reserves are exhausted, fats is the next nutrient your body oxidizes to provide energy for activities. Consequently, it plays a pivotal role in helping you meet your fitness objectives in a timely manner.

On this note, it is important to mention that oral consumption of essential oils needs to be done in extremely controlled quantities. The essential oils are concentrated essences of different plants. They have the capability to help increase your metabolism rate slightly or, in case a higher amount of essential oils is consumed, it can disrupt your digestive system. If excessively high amounts of essential oils are consumed, it may prove to be lethal as well.

The general rule of the thumb says you should begin by consuming a single drop of essential oil. It should always be consumed with a carrier like a drink or a meal. Its concentrated nature can harm your mouth and food pipe if consumed directly in raw form.

Once you figure out your body is tolerating the essential oil, you can gradually increase the quantity – drop by drop. However, make sure you do not increase the quantity too frequently or too much as both conditions can result in health problems.

Do research about the maximum quantity of essential oil concoction that should be used for weight loss. Make sure you never surpass this quantity as it then puts you at a disadvantage.

In case of external application or use of essential oils in soaking or bathing, the risk is substantially lesser. However, it is advised to test a small portion of your skin to see if the essential oil is well-tolerated. In case an adverse reaction is observed, consult a medical practitioner immediately.

Dilute the solution using carrier oils like jojoba and almond oil to decrease its intensity. It may help with eliminating irritation and rashes. Make sure the solution is safe for your use before applying it on large areas of your body. Consult your dermatologist to find out if there are any skin problems you have that may be aggravated due to essential oils.

Do not be in a hurry to adopt the trend – it may end up back firing. The use of essential oils is an intricate process that needs to be followed precisely in order to see the desired results. Otherwise, you need to be prepared for bigger problems!

Relaxing Your Way to Fitness

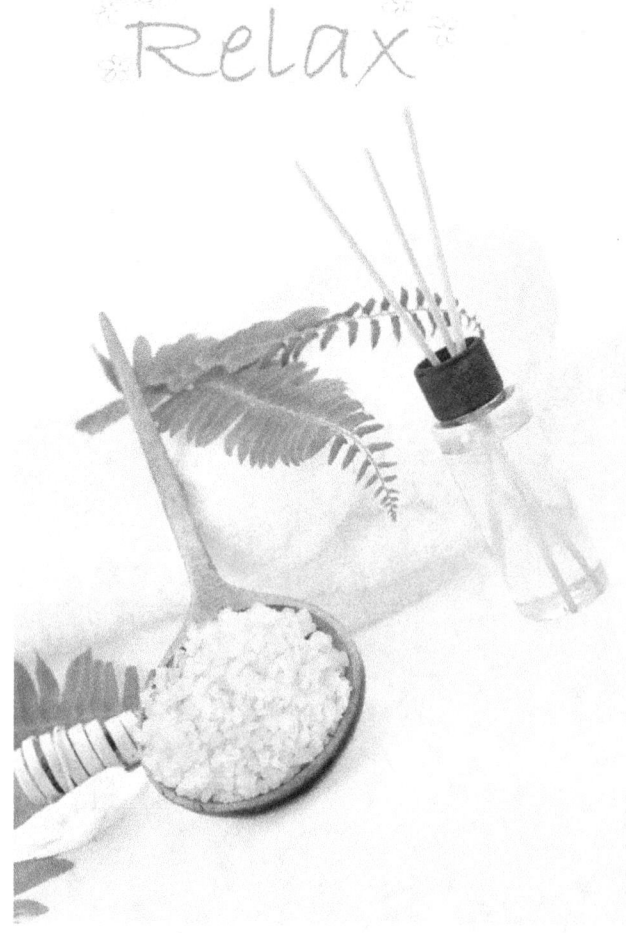

The use of essential oils for weight loss is a simple and effective feat. For the most part, you need not worry about stringent regimes or tiring gym schedules. It is easy to follow and quite effortless.

Using essential oils is painless provided you know when the quantity is enough. If you have sorted out this part of the equation (acquired the right tools to use for siphoning off the right quantity of the magic concoction), the rest will follow seamlessly.

If you look at it closely, you will notice that the use of essential oils is closely linked with stress relief. Soaking and bathing helps you relieve muscle tension and mind stress so you feel at ease. Likewise, external application involves a form of massage that achieves the same purpose. Inhalation and oral ingestion also trigger the same response in your body for same motives.

It is important to keep in mind that stress relief and weight loss are intricately interlinked. There are complex biological mechanisms working in the background that help you lose weight when you are not worried or stressed out. The hormones naturally produced and balanced in your body are attributed with this phenomenon. So naturally, you need to *relax your way into fitness and well-being*!

Essential oils help you achieve your goals by helping you relax and calming your nerves. In effect, workouts and healthy eating also restores your internal body balance with the same effect. Losing weight is not as difficult or tricky as it seems if you know what you need to do and how!

There are certain recipes of essential oils that can help you achieve your fitness aims in a timely manner. Certain combinations work better than individual essential oils.

Make the most of your time and resources – use essential oils wisely!

Health and fitness is just around the corner!

Recipes for Timely Success

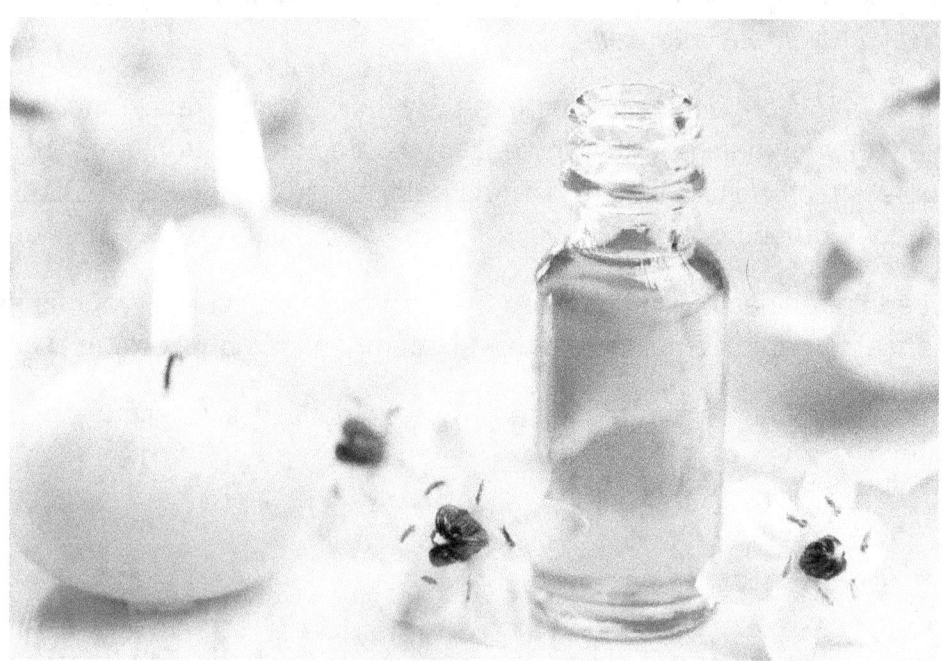

Here are some of the recipes of essentials that will help you in losing weight and achieving fitter, slimmer and attractive bodies in a timely manner. So here it goes!

The Grapefruit Remedy

Ingredients:

15 ml grapefruit essential oil

120 ml fractionated coconut oil

Method:

Mix the ingredients in a beaker and store in a spray bottle. This remedy is for external application only! After taking a bath, spray this remedy on those areas of the body that have high cellulite content and hence protrude from the natural structure. Use it consistently for the desired results.

Ingredients:

60 ml almond oil

0.25 ml or 5 drops grapefruit essential oil

0.25 ml or 5 drops lemon essential oil

0.25 ml or 5 drops cypress essential oil

Method:

Place the ingredients in a beaker and mix thoroughly. Store the mixture in a dark glass bottle. Roll the bottle lightly to mix the ingredients before use. Use a small amount of this mixture to massage your abdomen once or twice daily. You will begin to see positive results shortly.

Intestinal Ease

Ingredients:

5ml almond oil

0.05 ml or 1 drop of peppermint essential oil

0.05 ml or 1 drop of chamomile essential oil

0.10 ml or 2 drops of rosemary essential oil

0.05 ml or 1 drop of clove essential oil

Method:

Mix the ingredients carefully in a beaker. Store the mixture in an airtight glass bottle. This remedy is for external application only. Use a small amount of the mixture to rub the abdomen area in order to relieve intestinal problems.

Ginger and Grapefruit Surprise

Ingredients:

60ml of almond oil

0.45 ml or 9 drops of grapefruit essential oil

0.30 ml or 6 drops of ginger essential oil

Method:

Mix the ingredients carefully in a beaker. Transfer the mixture to a glass bottle for storage. Use a small amount of the liquid in your bath. The remedy is for external use only!

Ingredients:

2 ml of clove bud essential oil

1.75 ml of lemon essential oil

1 ml of cinnamon essential oil

0.75 ml of eucalyptus essential oil

0.50 ml of rosemary essential oil

Method:

Mix all the ingredients carefully in a beaker. Store the mixture in an airtight glass bottle. Keep in mind that this mixture is extremely strong and should be diluted before use. Ideally, add 6 – 12 drops of this mixture to 30 ml coconut oil before use. It can be applied externally.

Ingredients:

1 ml thyme essential oil

0.50 ml mandarin essential oil

0.35 ml clove essential oil

Method:

Mix the ingredients carefully. Transfer the mixture to an airtight glass bottle for storage. Dilute the mixture before you use it. Add 6 – 12 drops of this mixture to 30 ml almond oil before use. Alternatively, you can consume the mixture orally. Add a drop or two of this mixture to your drink.

The Internal Cleanser

Ingredients:

1.5 ml rosemary essential oil

1.25 ml lemongrass essential oil

0.5 ml thyme essential oil

3 barks of cinnamon

Method:

Mix the essential oils in a beaker. Transfer it to a glass bottle. Add the cinnamon bark making sure it is completely immersed in the essential oils mixture. Leave it to stand for two weeks before use. Dilute it with 60 ml almond oil before use.

Ingredients:

1.20 ml goldenrod essential oil

0.50 ml cypress essential oil

0.40 ml marjoram essential oil

0.20 ml ylang essential oil

Method:

Mix the ingredients carefully in a beaker. Transfer the mixture to a dark glass bottle for storage. Add small quantities to your meals to increase your metabolic rate slightly.

Ease Your Digestive System

Ingredients:

1.50 ml anise essential oil

1.25 ml rosemary essential oil

0.50 ml tarragon essential oil

0.40 ml ginger essential oil

0.40 ml fennel essential oil

0.15 ml blue tansy essential oil

Method:

Mix the ingredients carefully in a beaker and shift to an airtight dark glass bottle for storage. Add 2 drops of this mixture to your drink and ingest orally.

Ingredients:

1 ml chamomile essential oil

0.50 ml ledum essential oil

1.50 ml ylang ylang essential oil

1.25 ml geranium essential oil

0.75 ml sandalwood essential oil

Method:

Mix the ingredients carefully in a beaker and shift to an airtight dark glass bottle for storage. Add 2 drops of this mixture to your drink and ingest orally. It helps in relieving stress and emotional turmoil.

Energy Boost

Ingredients:

2 ml rosemary essential oil

1.5 ml balsam fir essential oil

1 ml juniper essential oil

0.50 ml nutmeg essential oil

0.50 ml peppermint essential oil

0.15 ml blue tansy essential oil

Method:

Mix the ingredients carefully in a beaker and shift to an airtight dark glass bottle for storage. Add 2 drops of this mixture to your drink and ingest orally. It revitalizes your mind and body so you feel active and confident.

Ingredients:

0.75 ml spruce essential oil

0.35 ml frankincense essential oil

0.30 ml blue tansy essential oil

0.10 ml rosewood essential oil

0.05 ml balsam fir essential oil

Method:

Mix the ingredients carefully in a beaker and shift to an airtight dark glass bottle for storage. Add 2 drops of this mixture to your drink and ingest orally. It helps neutralize energy and blood sugar levels for an active lifestyle.

Ingredients:

1.5 ml savory essential oil

0.50 ml thyme essential oil

1 ml lemon essential oil

1 ml raven sera essential oil

0.25 ml oregano essential oil

0.25 ml cumin essential oil

0.25 ml blue tansy essential oil

Method

Mix the ingredients carefully in a beaker. Transfer the mixture to an airtight dark glass bottle for storage. Add small quantities to your meals to ingest orally. It helps boost your immune system naturally!

Improving Liver Function

Ingredients:

1.5 ml Roman chamomile essential oil

1 ml ledum essential oil

0.40 ml German chamomile essential oil

10 carrot seeds

10 celery seeds

Method

Mix the ingredients carefully in a beaker. Transfer the mixture to an airtight dark glass bottle for storage. Make sure the seeds are completely submerged in the essential oils. Let it stand for two weeks. Add small quantities to your meals to ingest orally. It helps improve liver functions and keep its healthy.

Mental Peace

Ingredients:

2 ml bergamot essential oil

2 ml ylang ylang essential oil

1.50 ml rosewood essential oil

1 ml geranium essential oil

0.50 ml jasmine essential oil

0.25 ml Rose essential oil

Method

Mix the ingredients carefully in a beaker. Transfer the mixture to an airtight dark glass bottle for storage. Add small quantities to your meals to ingest orally. You can even use it to massage your head and forehead for the same results. It has a soothing effect and helps relax your muscles and nerves.

Ingredients:

1.50 ml lavender essential oil

1 ml roman chamomile essential oil

0.50 ml tangerine essential oil

0.25 ml citrus essential oil

Method

Mix the ingredients carefully in a beaker. Transfer the mixture to an airtight dark glass bottle for storage. Add small quantities to your meals to ingest orally. You can even use it to massage your head and forehead for the same results. This mixture can also be used in the form of baths and soaks.

Ingredients:

0.50 ml ylang ylang essential oil

0.25 ml marjoram essential oil

0.25 ml cypress essential oil

30 ml almond oil

Method

Mix the ingredients carefully in a beaker. Transfer the mixture to an airtight dark glass bottle for storage. Apply small quantities to your chest, hands and legs. Do not ingest this solution – it is for external application only.

Control Your Cravings

Ingredients:

1.50 ml tangerine essential oil

1.50 ml orange essential oil

1 ml ylang ylang essential oil

0.50 ml patchouli essential oil

0.20 ml blue tansy essential oil

Method

Mix the ingredients carefully in a beaker. Transfer the mixture to an airtight dark glass bottle for storage. Sniff the perfume heavily whenever you feel hunger pangs. The strong citrus smell has the capacity to trigger satiety in the mind so you feel less inclined to abuse your diet regimes.

Citrus Magic

Ingredients:

1.50 ml grapefruit essential oil

0.20 ml lemon essential oil

0.05 ml ylang ylang essential oil

1 teaspoon coarse sea salt

Method

Mix the essential oils carefully and store in an airtight dark glass bottle. Whenever you feel hungry or need to take care of your hunger pangs, simply add a few drops of this solution to the coarse sea salt and inhale heavily. The sea salt helps in retaining the essential oils for long so the scent remains intact.

Minty Magic

Ingredients:

1 ml peppermint essential oil

0.50 bergamot essential oil

0.20 ml spearmint essential oil

0.05 ml ylang ylang essential oil

1 teaspoon coarse sea salt

Method

Mix the essential oils carefully and store in an airtight dark glass bottle. Whenever you feel hungry or need to take care of your hunger pangs, simply add a few drops of this solution to the coarse sea salt and inhale heavily. The sea salt helps in retaining the essential oils for long so the scent remains intact.

Ingredients:

0.75 ml basil essential oil

0.75 ml marjoram essential oil

0.05 ml oregano essential oil

0.05 ml thyme essential oil

1 teaspoon coarse sea salt

Method

Mix the essential oils carefully and store in an airtight dark glass bottle. Whenever you feel hungry or need to take care of your hunger pangs, simply add a few drops of this solution to the coarse sea salt and inhale heavily. The sea salt helps in retaining the essential oils for long so the scent remains intact

Vanilla Inhaler

Ingredients:

1 teaspoon coarse sea salt

1 ml vanilla essential oil

Method

Whenever you feel hungry or need to take care of your hunger pangs, simply add a few drops of vanilla essential oil to the coarse sea salt and inhale heavily. The sea salt helps in retaining the essential oils for long so the scent remains intact. The vanilla essential oil in particular helps counter the cravings for sweets and baked items.

Ingredients:

1 teaspoon coarse sea salt

1 ml cocoa absolute essential oil

0.50 ml vanilla essential oil

Method

Whenever you feel hungry or need to take care of your hunger pangs, simply add a few drops of cocoa absolute essential oil mixture to the coarse sea salt and inhale heavily. The sea salt helps in retaining the essential oils for long so the scent remains intact. The cocoa absolute essential oil in particular helps counter the cravings for chocolates and other similar food items.

Abdominal Slimming

Ingredients:

0.20 ml lemon essential oil

0.20 ml peppermint essential oil

0.50 ml almond essential oil

1 empty capsule casing

Method

Place the essential oils in the empty capsule. Secure the lid carefully before shaking the mixture thoroughly to ensure the ingredients have mixed together well. Ingest the capsule with water or other drink of your choice. If stomach upset is felt, reduce the quantity of lemon and peppermint essential oils by half! Use one tablet per week initially. You can then increase the dosage to twice a week, thrice a week and then once daily. Do not consume more than one tablet per day to make sure no negative reactions are experienced. This concoction can help you lose roughly 10 pounds in about 2 months. It works exceptionally well on abdominal fats.

Ingredients:

1 bottle of grapefruit essential oil

Method

Carry the bottle in your bag or purse wherever you go. Sniffing the essential oil can help you combat hunger pangs. The citrus scent signals satisfaction to the brain so you feel less hungry and are therefore less likely to abuse your diet regime. At the same time, if you add 5-10 drops of grapefruit essential oil to a pint of water or some other drink, it will become a refreshing tonic. Use once or twice per day and witness the difference almost immediately.

Grapefruit essential oil is known to help increase the metabolic rate so you end up burning more calories in the given time period as compared with normal times. Do not overuse the product as it will lead to digestive complications. Use in small quantities only!

Ingredients:

1 bottle of peppermint essential oil

Method

Carry the bottle in your bag or purse wherever you go. Sniffing the essential oil can help you combat hunger pangs. The citrus sweet scent signals satisfaction to the brain so you feel less hungry and are therefore less likely to abuse your diet regime. At the same time, if you add 5-10 drops of peppermint essential oil to a pint of water, it will become a refreshing tonic. Use once or twice per day and witness the difference almost immediately.

Peppermint essential oil is known to help in suppressing cravings by signaling your brain that your appetite is full. However, do not overuse the product as it will lead to digestive complications. Use in small quantities only! Also, inhale heavily once or twice and then cap the bottle and put it away. Smelling the scent for prolonged periods will diminish its value in terms of being a hunger suppressant.

Ingredients:

1 bottle of bergamot essential oil

Method

Carry the bottle in your bag or purse wherever you go. Sniffing the essential oil can help you combat hunger pangs. The scent signals satisfaction to the brain so you feel less hungry and are therefore less likely to abuse your diet regime. At the same time, if you add 5-10 drops of bergamot essential oil to a pint of water, it will become a refreshing tonic. Use once or twice per day and witness the difference almost immediately.

Bergamot essential oil is known for its cholesterol reduction properties. It helps promote a healthier heart and hence a healthy lifestyle. It increases the metabolic rate and helps oxidize the fats in your body – even those that clog your blood vessels. Hence it can be used to promote overall health and well-being.

This essential oil can be used as an inhaler, an external applicant and also for ingestion. Be careful about the quantities of essential oils consumed to keep adverse reactions reduced to minimum.

Ingredients:

1 bottle of lemon essential oil

Method

Carry the bottle in your bag or purse wherever you go. Sniffing the essential oil can help you combat hunger pangs. The citrus scent signals satisfaction to the brain so you feel less hungry and are therefore less likely to abuse your diet regime. At the same time, if you add 5-10 drops of lemon essential oil to a pint of water, it will become a refreshing tonic. Use once or twice per day and witness the difference almost immediately.

Lemon essential oil is known to help in suppressing cravings by signaling your brain that your appetite is full. However, do not overuse the product as it will lead to digestive complications. Use in small quantities only!

Also, inhale heavily once or twice and then cap the bottle and put it away. Smelling the scent for prolonged periods will diminish its value in terms of being a hunger suppressant.

Lemon essential oils are known to help increase your metabolic activity and therefore encourage fat oxidization. So you can use it for multiple purposes to achieve a common goal.

Ingredients:

1 bottle of sandalwood essential oil

Method

Carry the bottle in your bag or purse wherever you go. Sniffing the essential oil can help you attain a sense of emotional balance. Much like other essential oils that are used individually, the sandalwood essential oil helps relax the tension and stress in your body. Consequently, you feel less inclined to abuse your diet plan or consume unnecessary foods under stress. It helps you follow your diet plan by helping you attain an internal body balance.

Sandalwood essential oil is known to help in preventing stress diets. However, it is important for you not overuse the product as it will lead to digestive complications. Use in small quantities only! Also, inhale heavily once or twice and then cap the bottle and put it away. Smelling the scent for prolonged periods will diminish its value in terms of being a hunger suppressant.

The Sandalwood essential oil can be used as an inhaler, as an oral ingestion (in the form of a drink) and also applied locally. Its basic purpose is to help relieve stress. Diet control comes naturally with this.

Ingredients:

1 bottle of fennel essential oil

Method

Carry the bottle in your bag or purse wherever you go. The fennel essential oil can be used in multiple ways including oral ingestion, external application and inhalation. The fennel seeds as a whole and the fennel essential oil in particular have been used for numerous health benefits. Apart from regulating hormones and helping in digestion, fennel is known to be anti-diabetic, anti-inflammatory, analgesic, antiseptic, and anti-microbial and so on and so forth. It improves digestion and promotes metabolic activity to help in weight loss.

You can sniff the essential oil on the go to help relieve stomach problems like indigestion and constipation. Moreover, you can also consume a few drops of fennel essential oil in a jug of water for the same benefits. Make sure you consume the essential oil in controlled quantities for best results.

Ingredients:

1 ml ocotea essential oil

1 ml lemon essential oil

1 ml tangerine essential oil

1 ml grapefruit essential oil

1 ml spearmint essential oil

1 teaspoon stevia (for sweetening if required)

Method

Carefully mix the essential oils in a beaker and store in an airtight dark bottle. Add a few drops of this solution to a glass of water and consume it orally. Alternatively, you can also apply the essential oils locally (without stevia) for the same results. This concoction is suitable for baths and soaks as well. Make sure you dilute the essential oils mixture before use.

The Tangy Special

Ingredients:

1 ml lemon essential oil

1 ml mandarin essential oil

1 ml tangerine essential oil

1 ml orange essential oil

1 ml grapefruit essential oil

1 ml spearmint essential oil

Method

Carefully mix the essential oils in a beaker. Transfer this mixture to an airtight dark bottle for storage. It can be used as an inhaler, an external applicant as well as ingestion. Dilute the mixture in a glass of water for oral usage. If you plan to use it as massage oil, remember to dilute this solution with at least 20 ml almond oil. Ideal for use near the ears, neck and feet areas. In addition to antiseptic properties, the essential oils have relaxing characteristics which help in inhibiting stress eating. It also boosts the body metabolism naturally for the same results.

Ingredients:

1 ml basil essential oil

1 ml sage essential oil

1 ml marjoram essential oil

Method

Mix the ingredients carefully and store in an airtight dark bottle. Keep it close by. Every time you experience a certain craving, sniff the mixture heavily for two seconds and recap the bottle. It will help lessen the intensity of hunger pangs.

Remember not to use this mixture over an extended time period as inhaling the combination too often will reduce its effectiveness. Use it for a week and ground it for two weeks before using again so that your brain recognizes it as a foreign scent!

Home Spa

Ingredients:

0.40 ml grapefruit essential oil

0.10 ml thyme essential oil

0.10 ml fennel essential oil

0.10 ml lavender essential oil

0.10 ml rose essential oil

0.10 berry essential oil

400 ml almond oil

Method

Mix the ingredients carefully and transfer it to a plastic spray bottle. The mixture works best when used after a bath. Once you have exfoliated the skin, use generous amounts of the liquid to massage your body. Take about 20 minutes to massage and then cover each area with cellophane to retain its effect. Let the cellophane paper stay for 20 minutes before discarding it. Take a final bath – first with warm water and then with cold water. Pat the skin dry and experience an elevated sense of relaxation! It is suitable for males as well as females.

Ingredients

0.25 ml lime essential oil

0.20 ml cedar wood essential oil

0.15 ml black pepper essential oil

0.40 ml cypress essential oil

40 ml fractionated coconut oil

Method

Mix the essential oils carefully and store in an airtight dark bottle. At the time of use, spray generous amounts of the oil on your body and massage for a minimum of 30 minutes. Let it stay for 3-4 hours before washing off. The essential oils will not only moisture the skin and make it smoother but will also help you relax muscle tension. You can use the mixture multiple times during a week or on a weekly basis for best results.

Essential Tea

Ingredients:

0.05 ml lemon essential oil

0.05 ml lovage essential oil

Juice of 1 medium sized lemon

½ teaspoon lemon peel finely chopped

350 ml bottle soda water

Method

Mix all the ingredients carefully in a container. Cool the mixture in the refrigerator before use. Ideally, this cold tea is to be consumed before breakfast. It does not only detoxify the body from all kinds of chemical hazards that you may have consumed but also freshens up the mind and the body for the challenges to be faced during the day!

Ingredients:

0.25 ml juniper berry essential oil

0.25 ml cypress essential oil

0.25 ml orange essential oil

Method

Mix the essential oils carefully and transfer to an airtight dark bottle for storage. At the time of use, carefully tip the contents of this bottle to a bath. Soak yourself in the fragrant liquid for 30 minutes. The oils help repair your skin cells so they can retain the moisture content in a better manner. You will immediately notice a significant improvement in the texture and feel of your skin following this treatment.

Improving Blood Circulation

Ingredients:

30 ml fractionated coconut oil

0.75 ml of essential oil (You can use birch essential oil, clay essential oil, sage essential oil, cypress essential oil, orange essential oil, rosemary essential oil, eucalyptus essential oil, or juniper berry essential oil)

Method

Mix the essential oils carefully making sure the solution has merged properly. Use the oil as required to massage your body. Generally, it is recommended to use extremely small amounts of the mixture to minimize adverse effects. The essential oils have the capacity to relieve edema and increase blood circulation in the body. However, do not consume this mixture orally. It is for external use only!

You can use the mixture to massage multiple times during the day. Leave the oils on for at least half an hour before washing it off.

Ingredients:

1 ml grapefruit essential oil

1 ml lemon essential oil

1 ml peppermint essential oil

1 ml ginger essential oil

1 ml cinnamon essential oil

Method

Mix the ingredients carefully and store in a dark airtight bottle. Keep away from direct sunlight and heat.

This mixture can be used for inhalation, external application, in baths and soaks. However, it is strictly not recommended for oral consumption. Dilute a few drops of this mixture in a tub of water before coming into contact with the solution. The essential oils in this mixture are very strong. Use in extremely controlled quantities to keep the negative effects of the solution to a minimum.

This solution contains de-stressing properties and can be used by males as well as females. Apart from this, the solution is known to revitalize the body, the mind and the spirit so you feel amazingly refreshed and energetic. In case you feel any sort of tingling or irritation, dilute the bath solution further with water.

Ingredients:

60 grams of cocoa butter

20 grams avocado oil

0.20 ml neroli essential oil

Method

Heat the cocoa butter slowly over a double boiler. Once fully liquefied, add in the avocado oil and stir thoroughly. Remove the mixture from heat. As the mixture begins to solidify, add in the neroli essential oil drop by drop. Mix thoroughly to ensure the solution is even. Transfer the mixture to a cosmetic container with a wide mouth and tight fitting lid. As it cools, the solution will solidify. Store carefully and use generous amounts of the "cream" to massage the problem areas of your skin. Works best on stretch marks and dry skins.

Ingredients:

60 ml almond oil or jojoba essential oil

1 ml roman chamomile essential oil

0.25 ml black pepper essential oil

Method

Mix all the ingredients carefully in a beaker and transfer to an airtight dark container for storage. Take a small amount of the oil and massage the affected area lightly. Use round movements for maximum impact. Do consult your orthopedic doctor before using this remedy as depending on your condition, your doctor might suggest a few specific movements to ease pain.

Try not to apply a lot of essential oil directly to your skin as the essential oils in general are quite harsh and strong.

Ingredients:

60 ml almond oil or jojoba essential oil

0.50 ml roman chamomile essential oil

0.50 ml helichrysum essential oil

Method

Mix all the ingredients carefully in a beaker and transfer to an airtight dark container for storage. Take a small amount of the oil and massage the affected area lightly. Use round movements for maximum impact. Do consult your orthopedic doctor before using this remedy as depending on your condition, your doctor might suggest a few specific movements to ease pain.

Try not to apply a lot of essential oil directly to your skin as the essential oils in general are quite harsh and strong.

Ingredients:

0.05 ml rose essential oil

0.15 ml orange essential oil

0.05 ml vetiver essential oil

Method

Mix the ingredients carefully in a container and shift to an airtight dark bottle for storage. Dilute it with 20 ml carrier oil such as the jojoba essential oil or the fractionated essential oil. It can be used for aromatherapy, for bathing and soaking as well as for massaging. Use the mixture of essential oils as per your requirement. You can also carry it around in your bag/purse and use it as an inhaler.

Agitation Rescue

Ingredients:

0.15 ml bergamot essential oil

0.05 ml ylang ylang essential oil

0.05 ml jasmine essential oil

Method

Mix the ingredients carefully in a container and shift to an airtight dark bottle for storage. Dilute it with 20 ml carrier oil such as the jojoba essential oil or the fractionated essential oil. It can be used for aromatherapy, for bathing and soaking as well as for massaging. Use the mixture as per your preference and requirement. You can also carry it around in your bag/purse and use it as an inhaler.

Ingredients:

0.05 ml rose essential oil

0.15 ml sandalwood essential oil

0.05 ml orange essential oil

Method

Mix the ingredients carefully in a container and shift to an airtight dark bottle for storage. Dilute it with 20 ml carrier oil such as the jojoba essential oil or the fractionated essential oil. It can be used for aromatherapy, for bathing and soaking as well as for massaging. Use the mixture as per your preference and requirement. You can also carry it around in your bag/purse and use it as an inhaler.

From Lows to Highs

Ingredients:

0.15 ml bergamot essential oil

0.10 ml clary sage essential oil

Method

Mix the ingredients carefully in a container and shift to an airtight dark bottle for storage. Dilute it with 20 ml carrier oil such as the jojoba essential oil or the fractionated essential oil at the time of use. It can be used for aromatherapy, for bathing and soaking as well as for massaging. Use the mixture as per your preference and requirement. You can also carry it around in your bag/purse and use it as an inhaler.

Relaxol

Ingredients:

20 ml carrier oil such as the jojoba essential oil or the almond oil

0.50 ml roman chamomile essential oil

0.25 ml lavender essential oil

Method

Mix the ingredients carefully in a container and shift to an airtight dark bottle for storage. Dilute it with 20 ml carrier oil such as the jojoba essential oil or the fractionated essential oil. It can be used for aromatherapy, for bathing and soaking as well as for massaging. Use the mixture as per your preference and requirement. You can also carry it around in your bag/purse and use it as an inhaler.

This remedy works best when you use it to massage your feet for about 20 minutes. Massage slowly applying balanced pressure on the pressure points in your feet. You will feel the stress and anxiety reducing so you feel relaxed and at peace.

Energize Your Day

Ingredients:

0.10 ml basil essential oil

0.05 ml cypress essential oil

0.10 ml grapefruit essential oil

Method

Mix the ingredients carefully in a container and shift to an airtight dark bottle for storage. Dilute it with 20 ml carrier oil such as the jojoba essential oil or the fractionated essential oil. It can be used for aromatherapy, for bathing and soaking as well as for massaging. Use the mixture as per your preference and requirement. You can also carry it around in your bag/purse and use it as an inhaler.

For best results, use this solution early in the morning for a truly energized day ahead!

Ingredients:

0.10 ml peppermint essential oil

0.05 ml frankincense essential oil

0.10 ml lemon essential oil

Method

Mix the ingredients carefully in a container and shift to an airtight dark bottle for storage. Dilute it with 20 ml carrier oil such as the jojoba essential oil or the fractionated essential oil. It can be used for aromatherapy, for bathing and soaking as well as for massaging. Use the mixture as per your preference and requirement. You can also carry it around in your bag/purse and use it as an inhaler.

For best results, use this solution early in the morning for a truly energized day ahead!

Ingredients:

0.15 ml bergamot essential oil

0.05 ml ylang ylang essential oil

0.05 ml grapefruit essential oil

Method

Mix the ingredients carefully in a container and shift to an airtight dark bottle for storage. Dilute it with 20 ml carrier oil such as the jojoba essential oil or the fractionated essential oil. It can be used for aromatherapy, for bathing and soaking as well as for massaging. Use the mixture as per your preference and requirement. You can also carry it around in your bag/purse and use it as an inhaler.

It is an ideal getaway from the problems of your day to day life. You can use it as the perfect beginning for a rejuvenating weekend.

Conclusion

The essential oils have multiple purposes other than simply serving as aesthetic scents. As evidenced throughout this eBook, the essential oils can be used to promote overall health and well-being which eventually plays a pivotal role in encouraging healthy weight loss.

It is important to keep in mind that essential oils will probably be insufficient in meeting your fitness goals if you do not employ the right practices when it comes to your diet and exercise routine. Nevertheless, it gives your regime an additional boost for quick and timely results.

The essential oils work internally as well as externally. Make sure you consult your doctor in order to identify any complication present with the use of essential oils. The rest should all be fine.

So what are you waiting for? Make steady progress on your pathway to health and fitness! We wish you all the best for the success of your fitness endeavors!